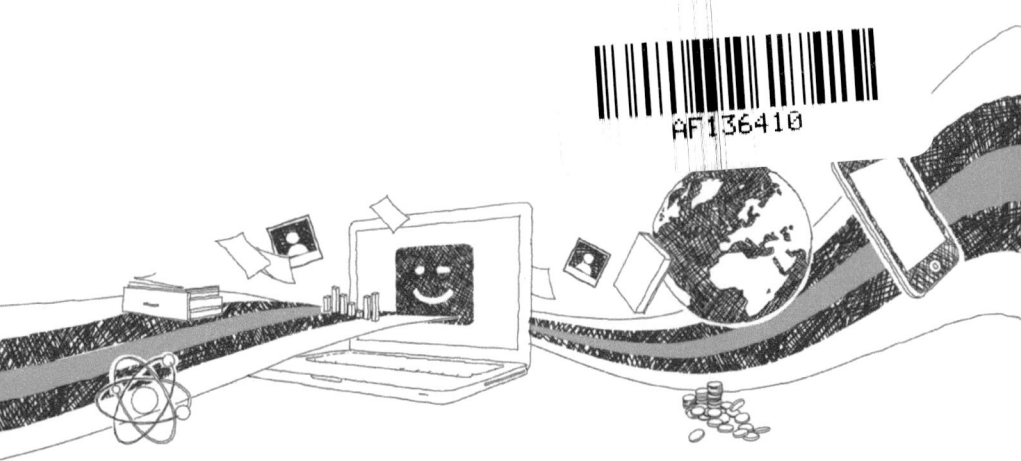
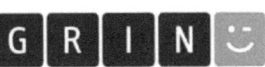

Bibliographic information published by the German National Library:

The German National Library lists this publication in the National Bibliography; detailed bibliographic data are available on the Internet at http://dnb.dnb.de .

Imprint:

Copyright © 2010 GRIN Verlag
Print and binding: Books on Demand GmbH, Norderstedt Germany
ISBN: 9783346067340

This book at GRIN:

https://www.grin.com/document/502602

Eddy Mihigo

The hand-arm vibration syndrome and the limits of construction workers' daily exposure levels of vibration

GRIN Verlag

GRIN - Your knowledge has value

Since its foundation in 1998, GRIN has specialized in publishing academic texts by students, college teachers and other academics as e-book and printed book. The website www.grin.com is an ideal platform for presenting term papers, final papers, scientific essays, dissertations and specialist books.

Visit us on the internet:

http://www.grin.com/

http://www.facebook.com/grincom

http://www.twitter.com/grin_com

Faculty of Health Sciences

Department of Environmental Health

Name: EDDY MIHIGO

Final Project Report

Research Topic:

A study of the daily exposure levels to hand transmitted and whole body vibration of construction workers in a construction site within the University of Botswana

Table of Contents

Acknowledgements

I would like to acknowledge the Department of Environmental Health for giving me the opportunity to carry out this monumental study. A special thanks to the Head of Department, Dr. R. Matchaba-Hove for his guidance, and to Ms Patience Tirelo for her patience and sound supervision.

Mr Simba, head of safety at the site of interest gets special mention for his support and cooperation, and the dedicated workers and labourers that provided the all important data get my thanks.

Most importantly, my family and colleagues are appreciated for the moral support and constructive criticism.

Abstract

Title of the project: A study of the daily exposures to hand transmitted vibration and whole body vibration in a construction site within the University of Botswana.

Introduction: Vibration is the oscillatory motion of bodies (Chaffin et al, 2006). It is divided into hand transmitted vibration, which is vibration entering the body through hands, and whole body vibration, which enters the body when it is supported by some vibrating surface. There are over 8 million workers that are exposed to vibration, and as an occupational hazard, it is not given much attention in Botswana and in most parts of the developing world.

Objectives: To determine the daily exposure levels to vibration of construction workers

Method: A quantitative cross sectional study design was used since there were different groups whose results were compared. The vibrometer was be used to quantify the daily vibration levels in each sample population, and the questionnaire distributed provided additional information as to the presence of symptoms or history of any discomfort resulting from the type of work. The population of interest includes the workers at a construction site within the University of Botswana, and these were divided into 5 groups, each group comprised 2 to 3 workers selected systematically, from whom data was collected depending on the tools available on the construction site. This means that the study population was 15.

Results: All the vibration levels were below the daily average exposure limit values, and the questionnaire was filled and answered successfully, with participants showing that they had basic information about vibration in general.

Conclusions: The objectives that were set out at the beginning of the study were achieved. The results suggest that the levels of vibration (both hand arm and whole body) are not high enough to cause any adverse effect to the workers. Furthermore, the daily average values for exposure is lower that the daily exposure limit values, which means that even after daily shifts, there is no adverse health effects from vibration from the machine. The questionnaire that was distributed assisted greatly in determining the participants' perception of vibration and its health risks, which can be said to be positive, although knowing about vibration does not mean one knows about how to reduce its effects.

Recommendations: In future, perhaps frequency studies can also be done, as vibration (especially hand transmitted vibration) occurs within a particular frequency range. Determining whether the participants are suffering from any symptoms arising from vibration should be considered in future, as it would be an indication that there is a problem, and action needs to be taken immediately. As for the organization, though they have solid administrative engineering controls that insist on job rotation every time one laborer finishes using the vibrating tool, it is also important to educate workers on the importance of personal protective equipment in lowering vibration levels (for hand arm transmitted vibration).

1. INTRODUCTION AND BACKGROUND

1.1 Introductory statement

Vibration is the oscillatory motion of bodies (Chaffin et al, 2006). It can be divided into hand-transmitted vibration and whole-body vibration. Hand-transmitted vibration is the vibration that enters the body through the hands (Gardiner and Harrington, 2005); and whole-body vibration occurs when the body is supported on a surface which is vibrating (Harrington et al, 1998). Hand Arm Vibration Syndrome (HAVS) is a group of symptoms related to the use of vibration tools (Sampson and Tonder, 2006). It is caused by the frequent use of hand-held tools over a long period of time. According to Burstrom et al., The quantity of absorbed energy is not only influenced by vibration intensity but also by several other factors, such as frequency, transmission direction, grip and feed forces, hand-arm postures and individual factors. The exposure limit values set for whole body vibration and hand transmitted vibration for daily exposures are 1.15 m/s^2 and 5m/s^2, according to the Health and Safety Executive control of vibration at work regulations of 2005. Shown below are values set for exposures according to 8 hour shifts.

The standards usually used for the measurement of vibration are:

- ISO Standard 2631 (1997) for whole body vibration
- ISO 2349 (2001) for hand transmitted vibration (Chaffin et al, 2007).

It is worth noting that some countries have their individual standards for measuring vibration.

Table 1: Exposure limits for Whole Body Vibration (8hr shifts)

Standard (Whole Body Vibration)	Time (hrs)	rms value (m/s²)	Health Effects
ISO 2631 – 1	8	<0.45	No major health effects anticipated
	8	0.45 – 0.9	Caution with respect to health risks
	8	>0.9	Health risks likely

(Adapted from Eger)

Table 2: Exposure limits for Hand Transmitted Vibration

Total Daily Exposure Duration (hrs)	Maximum value of frequency weighted acceleration (m/s²) in any direction
4 to less than 8 hours	4
2 to less than 4 hours	6
1 to less than 2 hours	8
Less than 1 hour	12

(Adapted from www.ccohs.ca/oshanswers/phys_agents/vibration/vibration_measure.html)

Vibration is measured in m/s^2, as the accelerometer measures the amplitude, frequency and exposure in all directions. There are also many tools used to estimate vibration, usually depending on what is being studied. This study focuses on the worker being exposed to the vibration.

1.2 Problem Statement

Research Question: Are the daily exposure levels of vibration to which construction workers are exposed within acceptable limits?

In 1974, NIOSH estimated that 8 million workers were exposed to occupational vibration in U.S industries (DiNardi, 1998). In Botswana and in most parts of the developing world, vibration is one of the least recognized ergonomic hazards, especially in construction. The few studies carried out have involved mine workers. For Instance, the first cases of Hand-Arm Vibration Syndrome were diagnosed in South Africa by researchers from the NIOSH who examined miners in a relatively warm mine (mean wet bulb temperature 28.6°C (Phillips et al, 2006). According to Sampson and Tonder (2006), the first documented research on HAVS in South Africa was a literature study written by Frantz et al. (1987). The objectives of the study were to determine the status of vibration-induced trauma in the mining industry, and also to give recommendations on preventative measure that could be taken before the condition became critical.

When one looks at its negative effects on the human body, which range from simple nausea to Hand-Arm Vibration Syndrome (HAVS), it is safe to say that vibration is not getting the attention it needs. Various technical developments in society have led to an increase in the number and types of sources of vibration to which people are exposed (Chaffin et al, 2007).

There are many facets of the local construction industry in which workers are exposed to vibration (both whole body and hand transmitted). Workers may see some symptoms of vibration such as tingling of the fingers (associated with hand arm vibration) and lower back pain (associated with whole body vibration) as a simple sign of fatigue, while in the mean time exposure continues and the problem remains serious. These symptoms also become more pronounced as exposure time increases, eventually causing disability that can range from being short to permanent. Those at high risk include workers that use machinery for more that one hour a day for hand held tools. For whole body vibration, older workers, and workers who may have a history of neck and back problems are mostly at risk. Looking at this, one can say that no one is safe.

1.3 Problem Analysis

The construction industry in Botswana has had a phenomenal growth, particularly in the last two decades. With the growth in the Construction sector comes a concern for the safety of the workers in the industry.

1.3.1 Hand-Arm vibration

'Hand-arm vibration syndrome' is a general term embracing various kinds of damage from vibration white finger, to neurological and muscular damage that can lead to numbness and tingling in fingers and hands.

Factors contributing to the risk of development of hand-arm vibration syndrome largely depend on both the magnitude of the vibration and the length of exposure. Some of these factors include:

- The grip, push and other forces used to guide vibrating tools or workpieces, (a tight grip transfers more vibration energy to the hand);
- The exposure pattern, length and frequency of work and rest periods (it is recommended that periods of exposure are broken up);
- How much the hand is exposed to vibration
- Factors affecting blood circulation, such as temperature and smoking
- Individual susceptibility

1.3.2 Whole body vibration

Whole body vibration is caused from vibrations passing through the body. It is a disorder that affects the lower back, spine, the neck and the shoulders.

Whole body vibration occurs due to various factors including:

1.3.2.1 Environmental factors

- Movement of wheels of vehicles and or mobile machines crossing uneven surfaces.
- The excavation of holes or trenches in the ground by the use of mobile machines
- The use of mobile machines for loading
- The hammering and punching of machines, crushers and compaction

1.3.2.2 Worker related factors

- Poor posture

- Long period of sitting in a single position

- Poor placement of controls which will need the driver to stretch or twist to uncomfortable positions

- Long periods of manual lifting and carrying of heavy objects

- Repeatedly jumping in and out of vehicle cabs

1.4 Justification

There are set standards relating to vibration such as; ISO Standard 2631 (1997) for whole body vibration and ISO 2349 (2001) for hand transmitted vibration (Chaffin et al, 2007). However, without the proper knowledge of the situation on the ground, it will be difficult to determine whether the standards are being adhered to.

There is no known evidence of any comprehensive study carried out locally that tackles the subject of vibration in its entirety. This study will offer information and recommendations on the dangers and effects of exposure to vibration.

The different industries that are affected by the issue of vibration are; building and maintenance of roads and railway, construction, estate management, forestry, heavy engineering, manufacturing of concrete products, mines and quarries, motor vehicles manufacture and repair, and public utilities (water, electricity). These will benefit from this study in the following ways:

- Economic loss reduction in the form of reduced compensation of workers suffering from disabilities related to vibration.

- Improved productivity in the sense that workers working in comfortable conditions will complain less.
- Reduced job losses. The lesser the number of workers that are disabled, the more the company's productivity is increased.

Lastly, the workers themselves will gain from this study by being informed about their health status and by being given information about how to prevent symptoms of HAVS and other complications related to vibration. They will be able to come up with programs for the prevention of HAVS symptoms at work.

2. LITERATURE REVIEW

Vibration is the oscillatory motion of bodies (Chaffin et al, 2006). It can be divided into hand-transmitted vibration and whole-body vibration. Hand-transmitted vibration is the vibration that enters the body through the hands (Gardiner and Harrington, 2005); and whole-body vibration occurs when the body is supported on a surface which is vibrating (Harrington et al., 1998). Although the two forms result in different effects, one can be exposed to both simultaneously. For example, when a jack-hammer operator holds the tool away from his body, supporting it and guiding it only by his limbs, he is exposed to hand arm vibration; however, if he leans against the jack-hammer with his abdomen, he is exposed to whole body vibration as well (DiNardi, 1998).

2.1 Hand Transmitted Vibration

Hand Arm Vibration Syndrome (HAVS) is a group of symptoms related to the use of equipment and tools that vibrate. Symptoms range from vascular and neurological to musculoskeletal, and affect different parts of the hand arm system (Sampson and Tonder, 2006). This is particularly important when it comes to hand transmitted vibration because these symptoms appear gradually, and become more severe with continuous use of the equipment. For some people, symptoms may appear after only a few months of exposure, but for others, they may take a few years.

2.1.1 Global Situation and studies

On a global scale, a lot can be taken as lesson from developed countries. According to Kaskosy *et al* (2003), in the USA 332 000 cases (of HAVS) were reported in 1994 and 305 000 in 1995 respectively. The cost of workers' compensation goes as high as 2 million American dollars.

In 2000, a study was carried out by researchers form the NIOSH who, according to Phillips *and* colleagues (2006), examined miners in a relatively warm mine (mean wet bulb temperature 28.6° C. The study involved 34 participants. 21 of these were re-assessed in 2004 to check the progress of their HAVS symptoms. Of the 11 (52%) who were initially diagnosed with HAVS in 2000, 10 showed progression. A second study was also carried out involving 21 rock drill operators from a cooler mine (Average temperature = 27° C). 52% of the volunteers in the cooler mines showed signs suggesting HAVS. This showed that indeed symptoms do get worse when unattended, and also reinforces the need for a study to establish whether workers are suffering from this condition.

2.1.2 Situation and studies in developing nations

In developing nations, the use of hand held machinery has increased with the increased development in infrastructure. Hand held vibrating tools have come into widespread use with the progress of industrialization in this area (Futatsuka *et al*, 2005).

In 2005, Futsatuka and his colleagues carried out a study of hand arm vibration syndrome among quarry workers in Vietnam. 50 quarry companies were selected for the study, and 73 operators were used with an average age of 31.2, and 29 workers formed the control group, with an average age of 33. Temperature was used as a factor to check for the recovery time of fingers after stress. Although the measurement was carried out according to

ISO5349-2, these were not explained in detail in the text. However, the study concluded that there was in fact a problem with regard to HAVS in the quarries. The inadequacy of this study proves the fact that not much is being done in developing countries to tackle the problem. The researchers seemed to have been in a rush to come up with results, which were not comprehensive. Furthermore, standards used were based on studies from developed countries. It is impossible to assess the impact of the labour situation on the health of workers in tropical areas because of lack of data from these areas (Futatsuka *et al*, 2005). With this in mind, it is therefore necessary to use standards from nearby areas such as South Africa as reference, as conditions are more similar.

2.1.3 Situation and studies carried out in South Africa

There has been extensive research regarding HAVS in the mining industry in South Africa, although most of the studies were carried out in the mining industry.

The first documented research on HAVS in South Africa was a literature written by Franz and others (1987). Franz *et al* gave recommendations that a study should be carried out to establish the status of the effects of vibration-induced trauma in the South African mining industry, and from this preventative measures could be developed before the condition reached an advanced stage. In 1999, Van Niekerk *et al.* (1999) carried out a study in which they were measuring vibration levels of different tools and equipments used in the South African mining sector. They were trying to determine the potential risk associated with the use of vibration tools, and also give some information on specific vibration tools and their health effects. From the study, it was concluded that the vibration levels on tools like hand-held rock drills, pavement breakers and jackhammers, were high enough to increase the risk of occurrence of HAVS. From this, it is seen that jack-hammers are related to occurrences to HAVS, which is turn related to excessive use of vibrating tools.

Another study then followed in 2002, carried out by Nyantumbu and his colleagues. This was the first epidemiological study on the prevalence of HAVS in Southern Africa. According to Sampson and Tonder (2006), in this epidemiological study the occurrence of HAVS was confirmed and a prevalence of 15% in rock drills operators at a South African gold mine was found. Nyantumbu *et al.* (2002) recommended that a screening be carried out in mine workers for HAVS. A suitable screening tool and questionnaire that are quick and easy to use and not expensive would be ideal if used as part of the annual medical surveillance of mine workers (Sampson and Tonder, 2006). This was indeed an in-depth study, as a screening tool was used in the form of a questionnaire. It could have been improved by getting information from the use of more tools.

Sampson and Tonder (2006) also carried out a study involving choosing the best way to screen mine workers for symptoms of HAVS. The screening tools chosen were a traditional tuning fork, a similar tuning fork but mounted into a box with a set excitation unit and a two-point discriminator set at 3mm, 6mm, and 10mm apart (Sampson and Tonder, 2006). The results showed that it was better to use a screening questionnaire that specifically focused on the symptoms of HAVS. Although the two-point discriminator with many different points of measurement was able to identify HAVS cases at 3mm, it had a lower sensitivity that the questionnaire. The study however concluded that it was best to use both methods.

2.2 Whole Body Vibration

Whole body vibration is shaking and jolting of the human body through a supporting surface usually a seat or the floor (HSE, 2005). In construction, workers usually blame lower back pain on fatigue, when it occurs as a result of whole body vibration.

2.2.1 Global Situation and studies

There have been numerous studies carried out in the developed world on whole body vibration. This may be because there are many industries in which machinery use is directly tied to low back pain symptoms, which in turn are directly linked to extended exposure to whole body vibration.

In 2006, Bovenzi *et al.* conducted an epidemiological study of lower back pain in 598 Italian professional drivers exposed to whole body vibration and other risk factors. A control group that comprised 30 fire inspectors not exposed to whole body vibration was also used. A structured questionnaire was also used to collect information on health histories. Alternative vibration dose was estimated for each subject from vibration magnitudes and exposure durations. Results showed a greater value of the 7-day and 12-month prevalence in the driver groups than in the controls. Furthermore, there was an increase in the occurrence of 12-month lower back pain, high intensity lower back pain and lower back pain disability with increasing cumulative vibration exposure. Also, individual characteristics such as age and body mass index were shown to be associated with lower back pain outcomes. The study confirmed that professional driving in industry is associated with increased risks of work-related lower back pain. According to Bovenzi *et al.* (2006), exposure to whole body vibration and physical loading factors at work are important components of the multifactorial origin of low back pain in professional drivers.

Once again in 2006 in Germany, Schust *et al.* examined the perceptions and reaction times during low-frequency vibration in x- or y- direction and biaxial (xy-) vibration of driver seats with activated and deactivated suspension. In this study, 12 male volunteers of weight range 59-97.7kg were exposed to whole body vibrations while sitting on the driver's seat, while randomly locking and unlocking the suspensions in the x- and y- directions. A brake and accelerator foot pedal had to be pressed on demand as fast as possible (Schust *et al.*, 2007). With a raised vibration magnitude, the intensity judgements increased and these were higher for the locked suspension, and the reaction times showed no significant influences of vibration magnitude, suspension or time.

In that same year, Johanning *et al.* conducted a study on whole body vibration and ergonomic study of US railroad locomotives. An assessment of the operator-related and ergonomic seating design factors that may have influence on WBV exposure and its effects was carried out. Measurements of vibration exposure were carried out according to international guidelines, and ergonomic work place factors and the effects of vibration were both studied using a cross-sectional survey questionnaire distributed randomly to 2546 railroad engineers and a control group. According to Johanning *et al.* (2006), the response rate was 47% for the RR engineers (n = 1195) and 41% for the controls (n = 323). This rate seems to be unreasonable, meaning that most of the workers did not take part in the study. This may have been because of lack of communication. Almost all the results were above the critical ratios found in ISO 2631-31 and the prevalence of advanced neck and lower back disorders among the engineers was found to be almost double of than of the control group without vibration exposure. When questioned, the engineers rate their seats as most unacceptable regarding different adjustment and comfort aspects, while the control group rated their chair more favourably. In a regression analysis, time at work with vibration interference was associated with an increased risk of lower back discomfort, shoulder and neck pains among railroad engineers. The researchers suggest that further investigations be carried out to improve cab designs to attenuate vibrations in the seats.

In 2007, Scarlett conducted a study for the Health and Safety Executive in the United Kingdom, in which the emissions and estimated daily exposure levels of whole body vibration on self propelled forage harvesters was evaluated. The study had as its objective the quantifying of whole body vibration emission and the likely daily exposure levels associated with the normal operation of self-propelled forage harvesters. A survey was also carried out to collect information concerning typical machine usage and operator perception of Whole Body Vibration levels. Comprehensive Whole Body Vibration measurements were made on 6 working machines, each encompassing 4-5 hours of commercial activity, to provide representative samples of Whole Body Vibration time-histories (Scarlett, 2007). In the results, whole body vibration levels were found to be moderate when compared to those encountered on other agricultural vehicles. Furthermore, vibration levels resulting form in-field harvesting were lower than those generated during on-road travel. From these results, a conclusion was reached that although the exposure action value (EAV) may be exceeded during normal daily operation, it is extremely unlikely that either the Whole Body Vibration daily exposure limit value (ELV) or the risk threshold will be reached or exceeded during a normal working day. From this study, the importance of relating the exposure action value to the exposure limit value is considered. It is also necessary to differentiate the two, something that was not done extensively in the above study.

Again in 2007 in the USA, Rahmatalla et al. carried out a study in the three-dimensional capture protocol for a seated operator in whole body vibration. A methodology based on using motion capture systems with reflective markers to detect position versus time motion of selective landmarks on the human body during vibration while taking into consideration the seat back was introduced in this study. By introducing virtual calculated markers that substituted physical markers, thus dealing with the fact that such markers (lower thoracic and lumbar section) could not be seen by the camera because of the seatback. The methodology was then tested on 3 subjects and there was considerable agreement between the physical markers and the virtual markers, and the results proved that the methodology may be useful in WBV testing. Though it seems that the study shows advancement in technology, it cannot be replicated as the exposure levels will be quantified in real time, and not modelled, as was the case in the above study. However, it is important to set up a standard methodology and protocol for the measurement of exposure.

2.2.2 Situation and studies in developing countries

In developing countries, there are many factors that affect exposure to Whole Body Vibration. As there is lack of proper infrastructure such as maintenance of roads and vehicles, exposure to Whole Body Vibration is worsened by factors such as the state of the road and tires, and the condition of shock absorbers and seats on the vehicles.

A study was carried out by Khorshid *et al* (2006) in Kuwait in which the main objective was to evaluate health risks associated with different geometry speed control humps. Vibration was measured following two standards; the British standard BS 6841, and the new ISO/DIS standard 2631-5. In the methods, effects of vehicle type, passenger location in the vehicle and hump geometry were also assessed. By using the two methods for measuring vibration, quality assurance was dealt with. The researchers came to the conclusion that all the aforementioned parameters had an effect on vibration exposure. The amount of shock that might harm the health of vehicles occupants depends on the vehicle speed, hump geometry, vehicle type, position of occupants in the vehicles, and evaluation method (Khorshid *et al*, 2006). This is critical, as it helps to consider all factors when evaluating vibration, especially in vehicles.

2.3 Concluding remarks

From the above, it is evident that there are several considerations to be made when evaluating exposure to hand transmitted vibration and whole body vibration. In the methodology, it is essential to consider two sets of standards for the measurement of vibration. This will ensure that a good comparison is made between the two. Furthermore, all factors that influence vibration such as position of the worker, state of the road, and more have to be addressed. It is also important to collect general information from the workers, this can be done with the help of a questionnaire or interviews, but it seems that questionnaires are preferred to interviews probably because there is no pressure to the worker (which would be otherwise provided by the presence of the interviewer) to answer the questions. However, most important is the communication of objectives to the workers as a whole, so as to remove any doubt as to what is being done.

There are challenges that are present, even with a near perfect methodology. Problems such as limited time to learn about the work environment before testing, poor control over the test setting, limited time for testing, poor cooperation, and lack of knowledge about vibration by health and safety people at the companies are some of the issues that make testing in the field challenging (Salmoni *et al*, 2007).

3. OBJECTIVES

To determine the daily exposure levels to vibration of construction workers

- To evaluate the awareness of workers concerning symptoms related to vibration (lower back pain and hand arm vibration syndrome (HAVS))
- To determine whether the exposure levels to vibration are within acceptable limits

4. METHODOLOGY

4.1 Study Design

A quantitative cross sectional study design was used since there were different groups whose results were compared. The vibrometer was be used to quantify the daily vibration levels in each sample population, and the questionnaire distributed provided additional information as to the presence of symptoms or history of any discomfort resulting from the type of work. The questionnaire will comprise structured questions which will provide answer options from the range of strongly agree to strongly disagree. The questionnaire was translated to Setswana, and there was a local on hand to help any of the workers answer the questions. This is where a great deal of help was required from the Safety and Health Representative of the organization.

4.2 Sample selection

The population of interest includes the workers at a construction site within the University of Botswana, and these were divided into 5 groups. These ranged from small power hand tools operators to office workers.

Table 3: Workers that participated in the study, the tools they use and their work description

Work description	Tool (equipment)	Number of workers participating
Small hand-held power tool operator	1 pneumatic drill 1 electric screwdriver	2
Compactor operators	3 light duty compactors 2 heavy duty compactors	5
Truck drivers	3 medium size trucks	3
Tractor operators	1 moving tractor 1 stationary tractor	2
Office workers	1 soft office chair 1 standard office chair 1 hard office chair	3

Each group comprised 2 to 3 workers from whom data was collected depending on the tools available on the construction site. This means that the study population was 15. Since the different groups yielded isolated results, a systematic method of sampling was utilized, where members of each group was selected depending on the number of available vibration equipment.

4.3 The HAVpro Vibrometer

For this particular study, the equipment that will be used was the HAVpro vibrometer, which measures both whole-body and hand-arm vibration.

The equipment was mounted on an adapter which was attached to the wheel. The accelerometer was then attached to the based of the adapter. This allowed for vibration to be measured in three axes (x, y and z). According to Eaton (2003), ISO 2631-1 requires measurement of frequency-weighted acceleration at the point of entry into the body.

4.4 Measurement for hand held tools (Hand transmitted vibration)

For hand held tools, the Accelerometer was connected to the hand of the worker as shown in the figure. For heavy tools such as heavy duty compactors, the accelerometer was attached to the wrist with a cushion.

The measurement method complied with the standards ISO 8041 and ISO 5349. However, there were few adjustments that were be made with regards to measurements of hand held tools. Because their vibration range was small, measurements were taken in decibels, and then converted to m/s².

Though these adjustments did not fully comply with ISO 5249, they helped in reducing some of the problems that arose with measuring vibration of light hand held tools such as constant mobility. To prevent this, the Accelerometer was tied to the finger that was used to pull the trigger on the tool. Vergara and colleagues (2007) carried out a study of hand-transmitted vibration in power tools, and found success with the similar alteration.

4.5 Truck drivers and forklift operators (Whole body vibration)

For whole-body vibration, a traxial accelerometer, which is inserted inside a rubber pad, was placed at the centre on the driver's seat. In all cases, it was important to ensure that all the axes were aligned as shown in the figure below, as per ISO 2631-1 requirements.

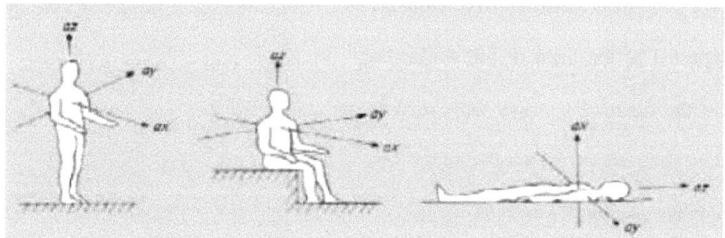

(From ISO 2631)

To ensure that data collected was representative of the natural environment of the drivers and truck operators, measurements were done while they were on-duty and along their normal routes. However, data was collected at one minute intervals and then extrapolated so not to intrude too much with the daily workings of the organization.

4.6 Additional calculations

4.6.1 Hand transmitted vibration

The values that were recorded in decibel had to be converted to m/s². This was done using the formula:

$$L_{dB} = 20 \, Log \, \frac{a}{a_0}$$

(Gracey and Associates, 2010)

Where a_0 is the reference acceleration values, which is 10^{-6}m/s²; and a is the measurement value.

4.6.2 Whole body vibration

The following formulae were used to evaluate the acceleration from all axes, for vibration for eight hours:

$$A_x(8) = 1.4a_{wx}\sqrt{\frac{T_{exp}}{T_0}}$$

$$A_y(8) = 1.4a_{wy}\sqrt{\frac{T_{exp}}{T_0}}$$

$$A_z(8) = a_{wz}\sqrt{\frac{T_{exp}}{T_0}}$$

(Griffin et al, 2006)

Where T_{exp} is the daily duration of exposure to the vibration (i.e. the Arms value) and T_0 is the reference duration (8 hours). The highest value of $A_x(8)$, $A_y(8)$ and $A_z(8)$ is the daily vibration exposure (Griffin *et al*, 2006).

4.7 Questionnaire

A questionnaire was filled by the participant after the data was collected, with questions relating to general knowledge about vibration and its symptoms, and whether any of the workers are experiencing any discomfort while using their various tools.

4.8 Ethical considerations

Before taking part in the study, the participant was asked to sign a consent form to ensure that he or she was not being coerced into taking part. The name of the participant was omitted from all documentations to keep his or her identity secret, and information from the questionnaire was not made public.

The organization was represented by the head of safety and health on the site, who helped in making the participants feel comfortable, and also supervised the data collection phase.

This study did not conclusively confirm that any discomfort experienced by the workers is directly related to the levels of vibration determined. Therefore, this study cannot and will not be used as evidence in any complaints regarding the relationship between vibration and discomfort.

4.9 Data management

The HAVpro vibrometer has an option that allows for the collection of data, calculation of results, presentation of calculated results and generating of a report. However, there were some manual calculations that had to be carried out. As mentioned above, the hand transmitted vibration daily exposure values had to be converted from decibel to m/s^2.

For the whole body vibration, the daily exposure values were not given, these values were calculated from the acceleration root mean square values using the formula above.

These values were then compared to the standard exposure limit values and exposure action values to determine whether the participants were being exposed to dangerous levels of vibration.

4.10 Data presentation

The data was presented in table form with the following variables:

Acceleration equivalent level (Aeq): this is the acceleration as it varies over a working day, measured in m/s^2.

Acceleration Root mean square (Arms): The weighted acceleration root mean square.

The vibration total value ($\sum$Arms): The square root of the sum of squares of weighted rms Acceleration (Deboli *et al*, 1999).

The daily acceleration value (A (8)): Acceleration recorded over an 8 hour period (or daily work shift)

4.11 Quality control and Quality assurance

Quality control was dealt with by the introduction of a control group. Also, because the vibrometer gave values that were pre-calculated, manual calculations were also carried out to complement and verify that there was no equipment error. Thus, the daily average exposure value for hand transmitted vibration was generated automatically; and the conversion to m/s^2 was done manually. The daily average exposure value for whole body vibration was calculated manually, but was directly measured in m/s^2.

For quality assurance, different standards and guidelines were used to validate method and analysis of the measurements; among them the ISO standards and the South African (SANS) standards. The equipment to be used will also be calibrated before use. The quality control measures stated above also contributed to the quality assurance of the study. These made sure that the study satisfied requirements for quality.

4.12 Limitations of the study

As with any study, this study had its limitations.

1. The sampling procedure: Since the sample population was selected systematically, there may have been some error attached to it. This may also be attributed to the fact that the population was small and based on available vibration tools.

2. Access to medical records: Access tor records is essential to establish whether really there may have been cases of injury related to vibration, or cases of HAVS. However the organization did not make this information available.

3. Reference Data: because this was a unique study in this area, there was no similar study to refer to for validation.

4. <u>Length of the study:</u> Vibration effects can only be seen over a long period of time. However this is a relatively short study that simply estimated levels on the ground, and whose findings were based on the information provided by the labourers.

5. <u>Bias:</u> because the study was supervised by the safety and health representative, the workers may have been scared to tell the truth. This may have introduced bias.

5. RESULTS

5.1 Pilot study results

Initially, the questionnaire was piloted to check for its validity. Five workers were handed the questionnaires, and these were returned the next day.

> **General Knowledge of vibration:**

- o Two of the five questionnaires **(40%)** answered showed confusion in answering questions five and six.
- o Of the five, one questionnaire was in Setswana, and the participant could not understand question eight.

> **Presence of symptoms:**

- o Four out of five questionnaires **(90%)** answered showed confusion with distinguishing between agree and strongly agree, and disagree and strongly disagree options.

5.2 Main study results

5.2.1 Questionnaire

Age of participants

Table 4: The age of workers that took part in the study

Age	Frequency
18 -24	3
25 - 31	7
32 - 38	3
39 - 45	2
>45	0

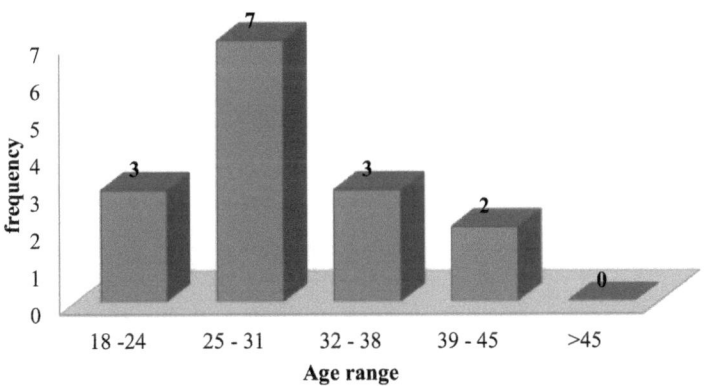

Figure 1. Age of workers that took part in the study

Gender of participants

Table 2: Gender of workers that took part in the study

Gender	Frequency
Male	14
female	1

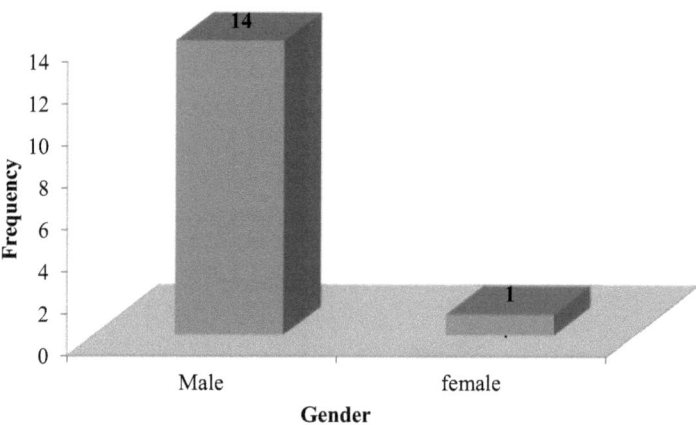

Gender of workers in the study

Figure 2. Graph showing the gender of workers that took part in the study. The single female worker was an office worker.

Perception to vibration

Table 3: Workers who have heard about vibration

Description	yes	no
Office workers	2	1
Tractor operators	1	1
Drivers	3	0
heavy duty compactor operator	2	0
Light duty compactor operator	2	1
small power tools	1	1

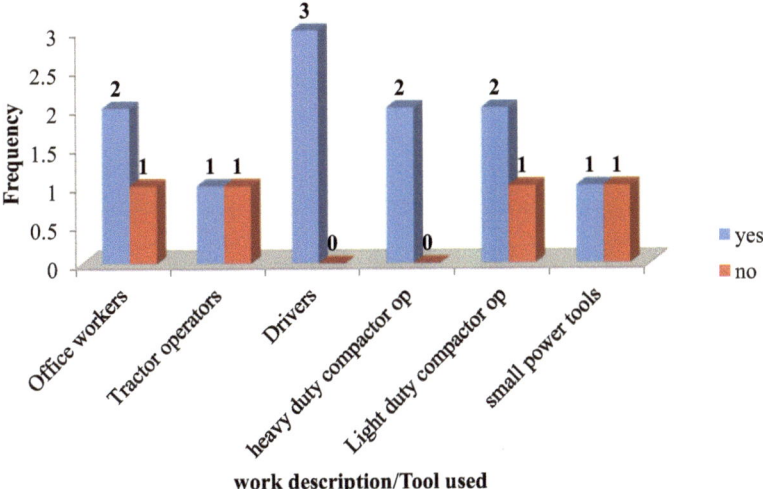

Figure 3. Graph showing the number of workers that said they had heard about vibration. The blue bar represents the workers that answered positively (yes), and the red bar represents workers that answered negatively (No)

Table 4: Workers who feel comfortable using their tools

	yes	no
Office Workers	3	0
Tractor operators	0	2
Drivers	2	1
heavy duty compactor operator	1	1
Light duty compactor operator	1	2
Small power tools	0	2

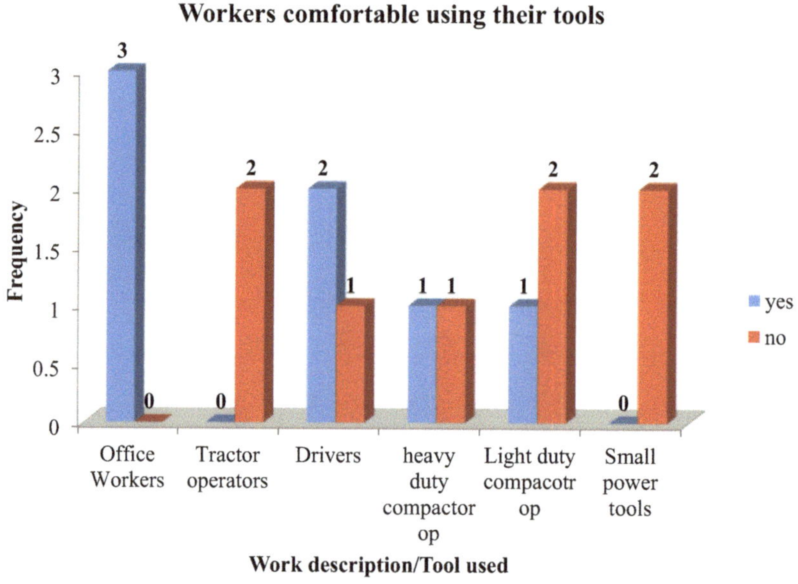

Figure 4. Graph showing the worker who said they felt comfortable using their tools.

Table 5: Workers who believe their tools make them feel uncomfortable

	yes	no	N/A
Office Workers	0	0	3
Tractor operators	1	1	0
Drivers	1	0	2
heavy duty compactor operator	1	0	1
Light duty compactor operator	2	0	1
Small power tools	2	0	0

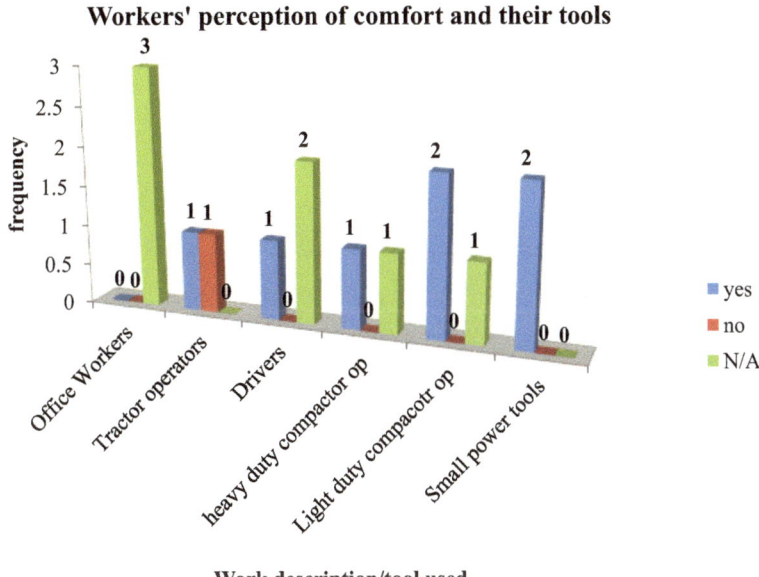

Figure 5: Graph showing workers who said they felt their lack of comfort was caused by their tools. The green bar shows the workers for whom this question did not apply, those who answered the preceding question positively.

Table 6: Workers who know that there is a relationship between pain in fingers and vibration

	Yes	No
Office Workers	1	2
Tractor operators	1	1
Drivers	3	0
heavy duty compactor operator	1	1
Light duty compactor operator	3	0
Small power tools	1	0

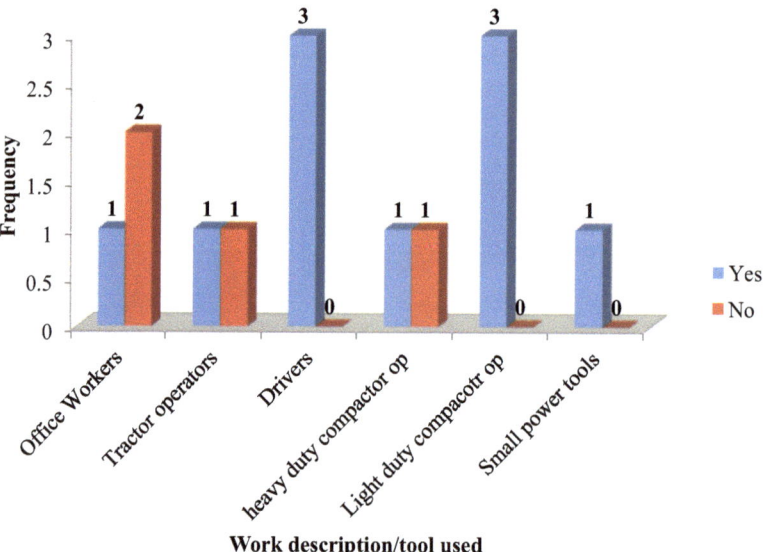

Figure 6: Graph showing workers who said that they knew that there is a relationship between vibration and pain in fingers.

Table 7: Workers who know that there is a relationship between back pain and vibration

	Yes	No
Office Workers	1	2
Tractor operators	1	1
Drivers	3	0
heavy duty compactor operator	1	1
Light duty compactor operator	3	0
Small power tools	0	2

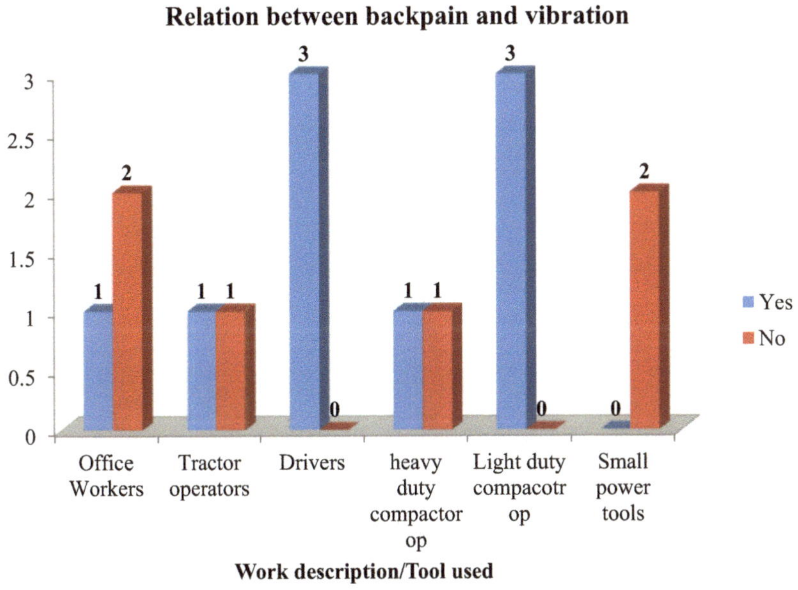

Figure 7: Graph showing workers who said that they knew that there is a relationship between vibration and back pain.

Presence of symptoms

Table 8: Workers who say they work more than 8 hours

	Strongly Disagree	Disagree	Not Sure	Agree	Strongly Agree
Office Workers	0	1	0	2	0
Tractor operators	0	2	0	0	0
Drivers	1	1	0	1	0
heavy duty compactor op	0	0	0	0	2
Light duty compactor op	0	0	0	0	3
Small power tools	0	0	0	1	1

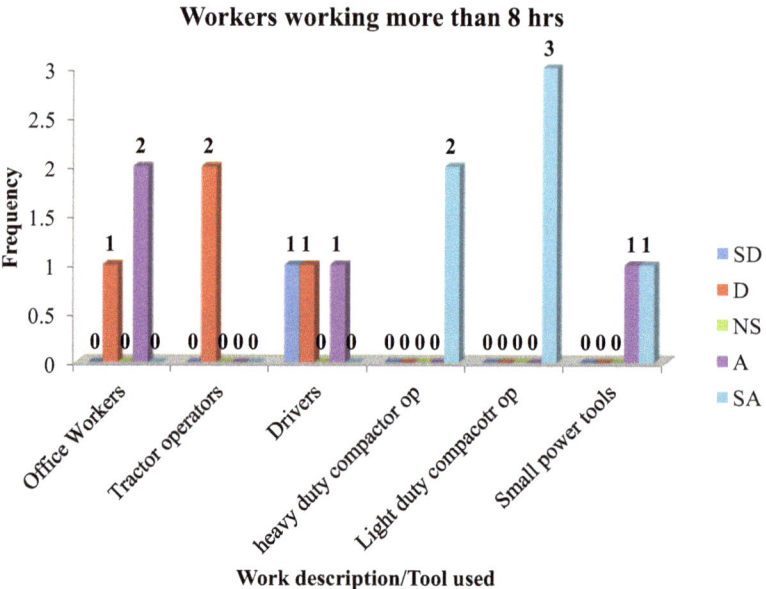

Figure 8: The graph shows workers' reply to whether they work more than 8 hours a day

Table 9: Workers who say they feel pain in their lower backs after work

	Strongly Disagree	Disagree	Not Sure	Agree	Strongly Agree
Office Workers	0	0	1	2	0
Tractor operators	0	0	0	1	1
Drivers	1	1	0	1	0
heavy duty compactor op	0	0	0	0	2
Light duty compacotr op	0	1	0	0	2
Small power tools	2	0	0	0	0
	3	2	1	4	5

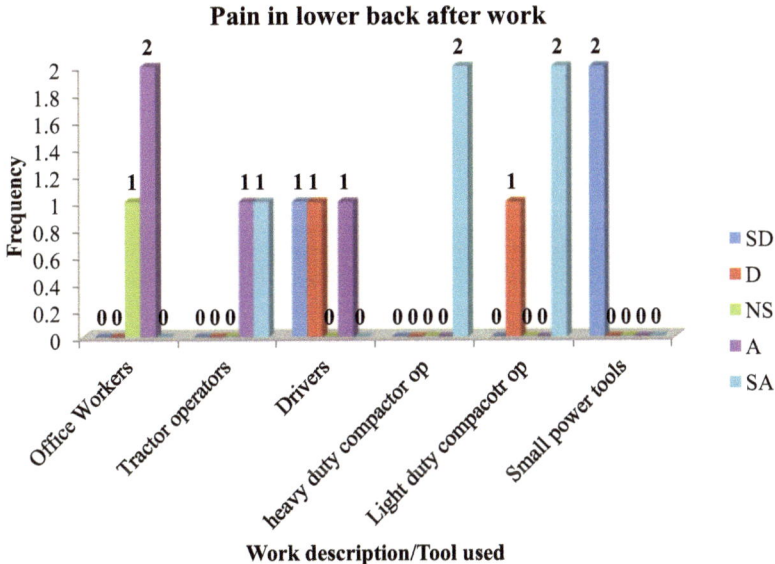

Figure 9: Workers' reply to whether they feel pain in their lower backs after work

Table 10: Workers who say they feel pain in their fingers after work

	Strongly Disagree	Disagree	Not Sure	Agree	Strongly Agree
Office Workers	1	1	0	0	1
Tractor operators	1	1	0	0	0
Drivers	3	0	0	0	0
heavy duty compactor op	0	1	0	0	1
Light duty compactor op	0	0	0	0	3
Small power tools	0	0	0	1	1

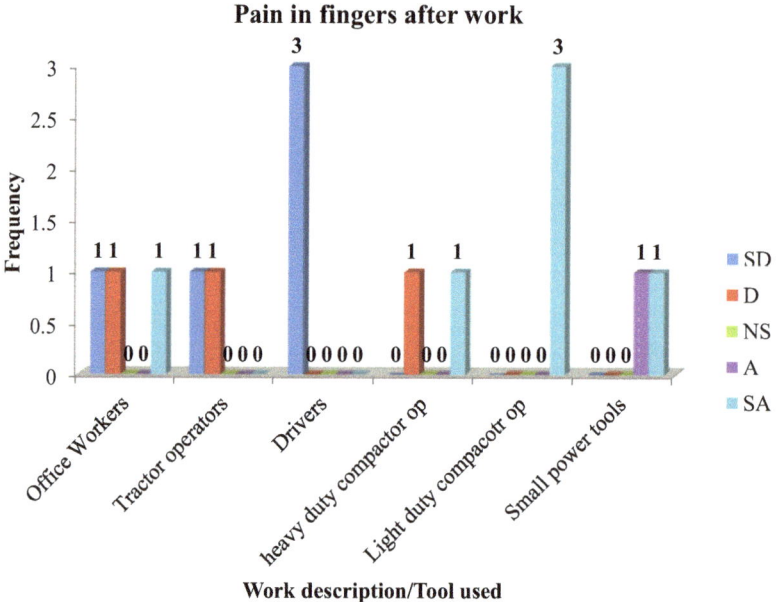

Figure 10: Workers' reply to whether they feel pain in their fingers after work

Table 11: Workers who say they feel pain in the neck after work

	Strongly Disagree	Disagree	Not Sure	Agree	Strongly Agree
Office Workers	0	1	0	2	0
Tractor operators	1	1	0	0	0
Drivers	2	1	0	0	0
Heavy duty compactor op	0	1	0	0	1
Light duty compactor op	0	1	0	0	2
Small power tools	2	0	0	0	0

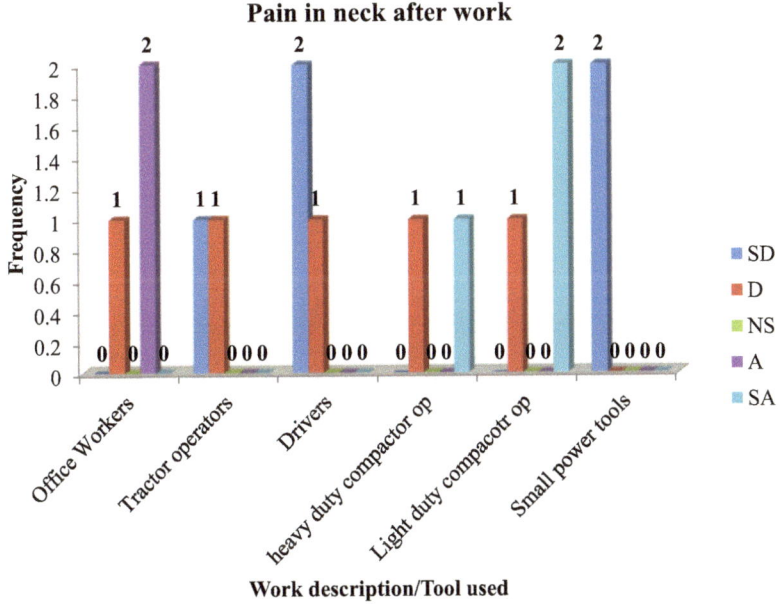

Figure 11: Workers' reply to whether they feel pain in the neck after work

Table 12: Workers who say they feel discomfort during work

	Strongly Disagree	Disagree	Not Sure	Agree	Strongly Agree
Office Workers	0	1	0	2	0
Tractor operators	1	1	0	0	0
Drivers	3	0	0	0	0
heavy duty compactor operator	0	0	0	1	1
Light duty compactor operator	1	1	0	0	1
Small power tools	1	0	0	0	1
	6	3		3	3

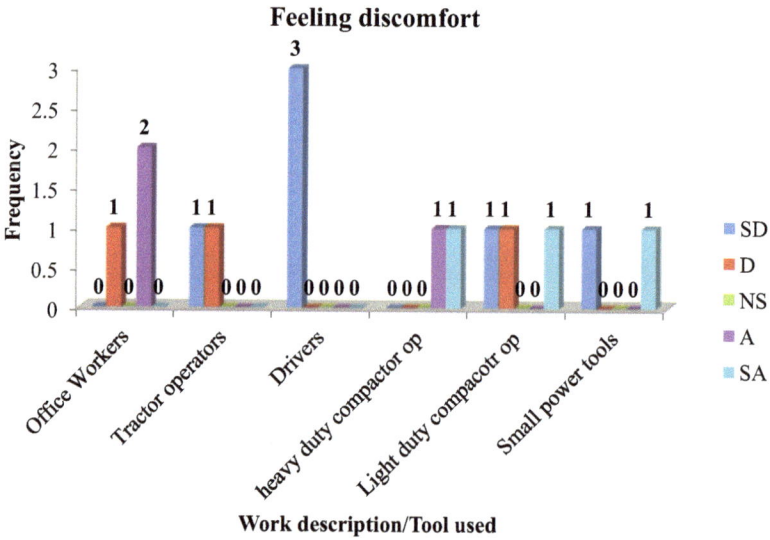

Figure 12: Workers' reply to whether they feel discomfort during work

5.2.2 Data analysis

5.2.2.1 Hand transmitted vibration

Table 13: Unconverted data

Tool being used	Arms (dB)	(actual) dB	Aeq (dB)	(actual) dB	A(8) (dB)	(actual) dB
Electric screwdriver	70	74.1	80	80	50	53.2
Electric drill	80	80.2	80	80.1	50	53.3
Light duty compactor 1	80	86.3	80	86	60	59.1
Light duty compactor 2	80	86.4	80	87.1	60	60.3
Light duty compactor 3	70	71	80	82.2	60	55.4
Heavy duty compactor 1	80	86.8	80	84.4	60	57.6
Heavy duty compactor 2	70	72.5	80	80.8	50	54

Table 14: Data converted to m/s^2

Tool being used	Arms (m/2)	Aeq (m/s2)	A(8) (m/s2)
Electric screwdriver	0.004	0.01	0.0004
Electric drill	0.01	0.01	0.0004
Light duty compactor 1	0.01	0.01	0.001
Light duty compactor 2	0.01	0.01	0.001
Light duty compactor 3	0.004	0.01	0.001
Heavy duty compactor 1	0.01	0.01	0.001
Heavy duty compactor 2	0.004	0.01	0.0004

Table 15: Daily A (8) compared to standard 8 hour ELVs and 8 hour EAVs

Tool being used	8 hour Exposure limit value (ELV) (m/s²)	8 hour exposure action value (EAV) (m/s²)	A(8) (m/s²)
Electric screwdriver	5	2.5	0.0004
Electric drill	5	2.5	0.0004
Light duty compactor 1	5	2.5	0.001
Light duty compactor 2	5	2.5	0.001
Light duty compactor 3	5	2.5	0.001
Heavy duty compactor 1	5	2.5	0.001
Heavy duty compactor 2	5	2.5	0.0004

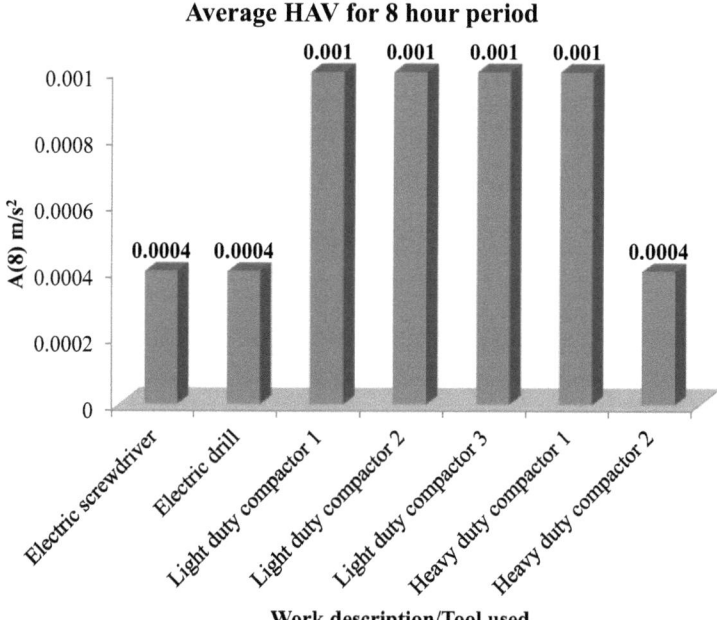

Figure 13. The graph shows the 8 hour average hand transmitted vibration values.

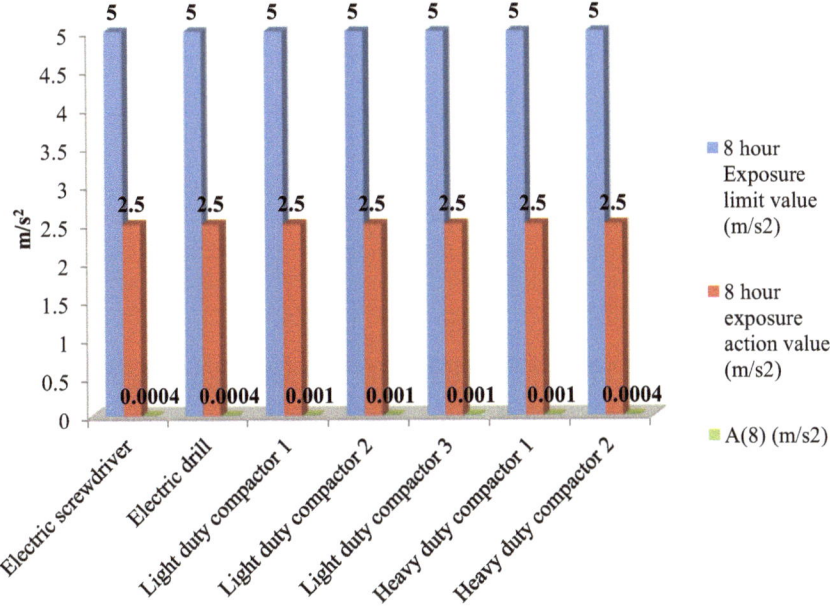

Figure 14. The graph shows the 8 hour average hand transmitted vibration values compared with the standard 8 hour exposure limit value of 4 m/s^2

Note: Raw data have been placed in the appendix.

5.2.2.2 Whole body vibration

Table 16: Average Whole body vibration daily exposure (A (8)) (Type of work)

Work description	Arms (m/s2)	A(8) (m/s2)	Av. Time worked (hrs)	Direction
Office worker 1	0.00994	0.0098	4	Z
Office worker 2	0.0694	0.0049	4	Y
Office worker 3	0.1760	0.0124	4	Z
Tractor operator 1	0.0161	0.0114	4	X
Tractor operator 2	0.0149	0.0148	4	Z
Truck driver 1	0.0194	0.0192	4	X
Truck driver 2	0.0769	0.1141	9	Y
Truck driver 3	0.0894	0.0885	4	Y

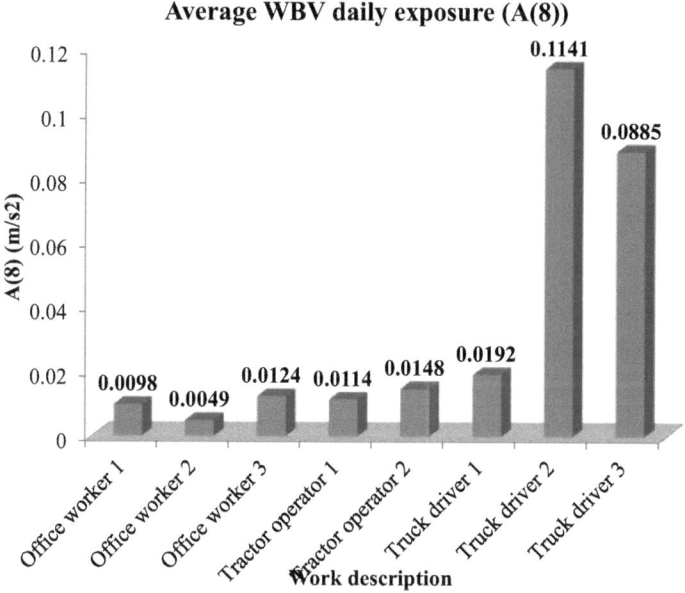

Figure 15. The graph shows average Whole body vibration daily exposure (A (8))

Table 17: Daily WBV exposures against standard exposure limit values

Work description	Standard values (m/s2)	A(8) (m/s2)
Office worker 1	0.315	0.0098
Office worker 2	0.315	0.0049
Office worker 3	0.315	0.0124
Tractor operator 1	0.315	0.0114
Tractor operator 2	0.315	0.0148
Truck driver 1	0.315	0.0192
Truck driver 2	0.315	0.1141
Truck driver 3	0.315	0.0885

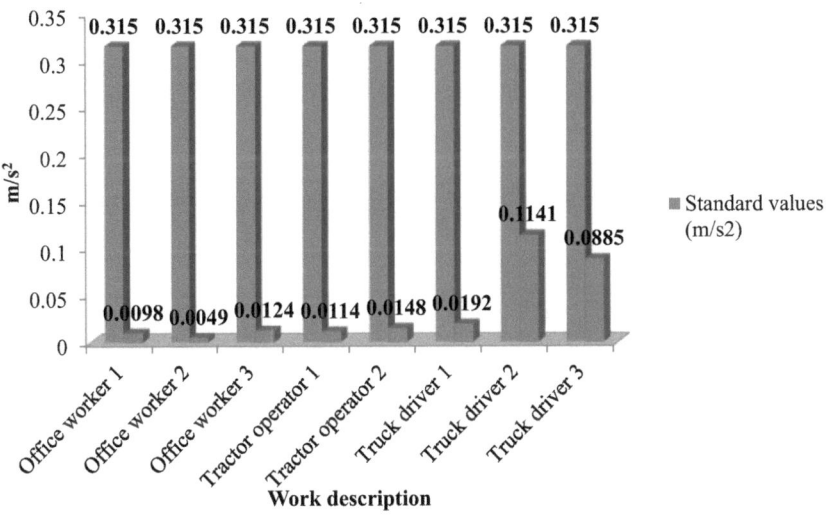

Figure 16. Graph showing average WBV daily exposures against ELV value

Table 18: Whole body vibration daily exposure (A (8)) (Equipment/Vehicle type)

Equipment /Vehicle type)	Arms (m/s2)	A(8) (m/s2)	Av. Time worked (hrs)	Direction
Soft cushion office chair	0.00994	0.0098	4	Z
Standard office chair	0.0694	0.0049	4	Y
Hard bottom off. Chair	0.1760	0.0124	4	Z
Medium duty tractor	0.0161	0.0114	4	X
Heavy duty tractor	0.0149	0.0148	4	Z
Light truck (tipper)	0.0194	0.0192	4	Z
Medium size truck	0.0769	0.1141	9	Y
Heavy duty (large) truck	0.0894	0.0885	4	Y

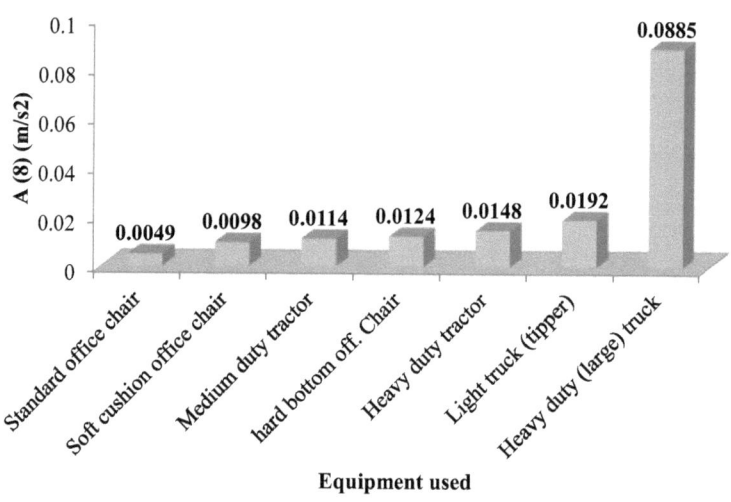

Figure 17: Graph showing the average WBV daily exposure (A (8)) based on equipment used

Table 19: Whole body vibration daily exposure (A (8)) (Equipment/Vehicle type) against lower ELVs.

Equipment /Vehicle type)	Standard values (m/s2)	A(8) (m/s2)
Soft cushion office chair	0.315	0.0098
Standard office chair	0.315	0.0049
hard bottom off. Chair	0.315	0.0124
Medium duty tractor	0.315	0.0114
Heavy duty tractor	0.315	0.0148
Light truck (tipper)	0.315	0.0192
Medium size truck	0.315	0.1141
Heavy duty (large) truck	0.315	0.0885

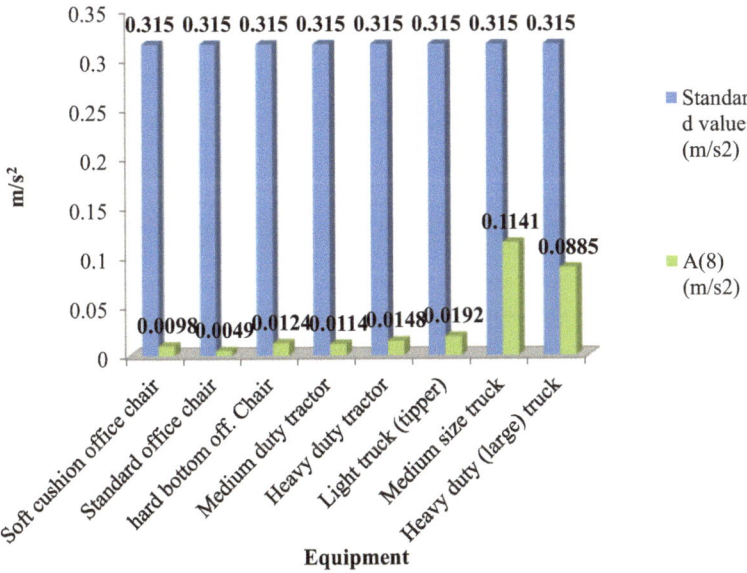

Figure 18: The graph shows the average WBV daily exposure against lowest ELVs.

6. DISCUSSION OF RESULTS

6.1 Pilot study

> **General knowledge of vibration:**

- o With two of the five questionnaires given out returning confusion, and one being difficult to answer because of language, it was determined that a different approach was to be used. One that would help the workers understand questions being answered.

> **Presence of symptoms:**

- o To deal with the issue of confusion with distinguishing between different options, it was decided that one of the workers would help in explaining some of the terms.

Based on these two major areas of confusion, it was conclusively decided therefore that interviews must be carried out before the questionnaire is administered; and that it must be completed and collected on site, so as to help with any arising confusion. The questionnaire was not altered in anyway however, as the questions themselves did not cause much confusion, but rather the participants' perception of the context in which it was asked.

6.2.1 Main study

6.1.1 Questionnaire

Age of participants

  The highest frequency of workers on site was those of the age range 25 to 31 (**46.7%**), and there were no workers above the age of 45. This may be attributed to the type of equipment that was being handled, though there was no particular relationship that could be seen between the age of workers and the type of job.

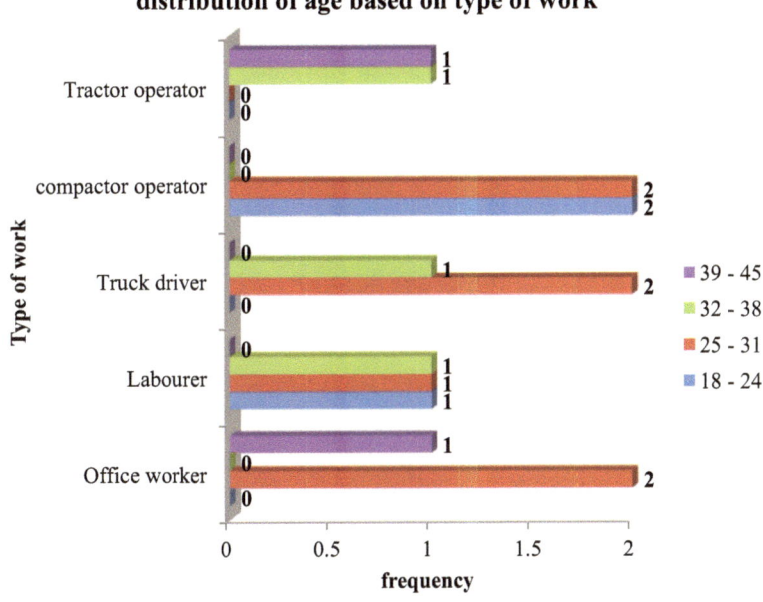

Figure 19: The graph shows the distribution the age of workers based on the type of job being carried out.

As can be seen in the graph, though the younger workers (age ranges 18 – 24 and 25 – 31) have the jobs of compacting, which require handling of heavy equipment, the older workers do not have any easy type of job. It can be seen however is that the older workers have the jobs that require a lot of experience (operating a tractor).

Perception of workers to vibration

Workers who have heard about vibration

Percentage of workers that have heard about vibration

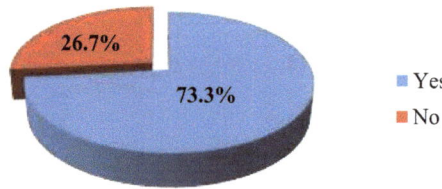

Figure 20: Pie chart showing the percentage of workers who said they had heard about vibration.

It can be seen above that a higher percentage of workers have heard about vibration in general.

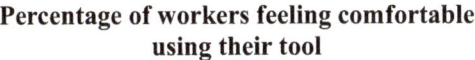

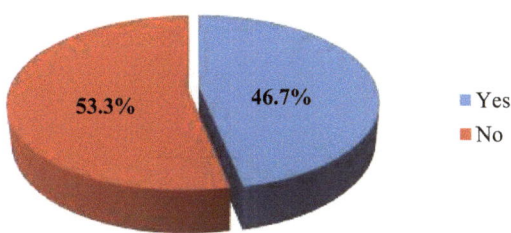

Figure 21: Pie chart showing the percentage of workers who said they felt comfortable using their equipment.

With the two answers being fairly equal, it could not be determined what may have caused this response. It could have been due to the equipment especially for workers using heavy duty compactors. However, some tractor operators and drivers said they were not comfortable. This may have been due to awkward posture caused by the type of seat being used. This also seems to be the view of Gustafson-Soderman (1987), who carried out a study in which he tested different types of seats of crane operators, and found that the highest estimated discomfort values were obtained from operators using the ordinary seat and the lowest discomfort values were obtained from use of the test seat with an adjustable sitting angle.

Therefore, the level of comfort could not be attributed to vibration alone.

Workers' perception of comfort and their tools

Percentage of workers who feel their tools make them uncomfortable

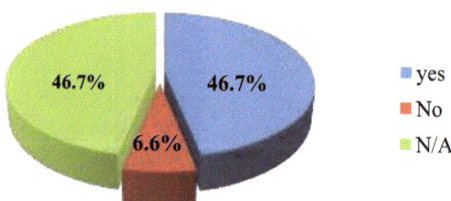

Figure 22: The pie chart shows the percentage of workers that felt their tools (chairs, compactors, small power tools). The N/A (not applicable) indicates the percentage of workers for which this question did not apply (those that answered the previous question positively).

The fact that 6.6% of workers felt that another factor caused them to feel uncomfortable strengthens the view that there must have been another contributing factor (such as awkward posture) apart from vibration that made these participants feel uncomfortable.

Bonvenzi and Betta (1994), who carried out a similar study found a linear trend of increasing prevalence of lower back pain (LBP) among tractor drivers that had an increasing perceived postural load. The study also revealed that tractor drivers with **excessive WBV and postural stress** had more than a three-fold increasing risk for chronic LBP than the unexposed subjects. This agrees with the view of the **6.6%**, who believed that there was another factor that caused them to feel uncomfortable.

Workers' perception of vibration and pain in fingers

Percentage of workers who know the relationship between pain in fingers and vibration

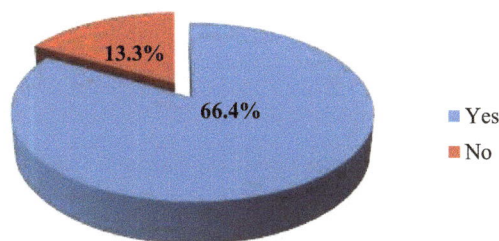

Figure 23: Pie chart showing the percentage of workers who said they knew that there was a relationship between pain in fingers and vibration.

Workers' perception of vibration and back pain

Percentage of workers who know the relationship between backpain and vibration

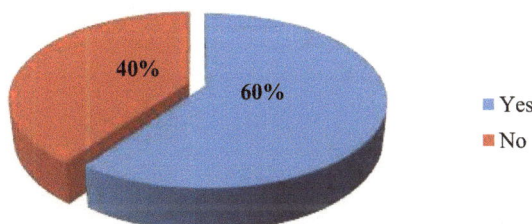

Figure 24: Pie chart showing workers who said they knew that there is a relationship between back pain and vibration

It can be seen that a large majority of the workers that were interviewed indeed did know that there was a relationship between vibration and pain in fingers **(66.4%)**, and vibration and back pain **(60%)**.

In a study that was carried out by Vergara and his colleagues in 2007, it was found that in 30% of the 216 interviews, 26% of those on which vibration was measured felt they were being subjected to excessive vibration. This fact tends to support the fact that workers do know what vibration is as they know when they are subjected to it.

Conversely, the same study revealed that workers are not really aware of the levels of vibration transmitted to their hands (Vergara *et al*, 2007). This was due to the fact that certain levels which were below $3m/s^2$ were perceived to be excessive. Therefore, while the workers do have general information about vibration, they have no way of detecting when levels are excessive or not.

The fact that the workers know of the relationship between vibration and back pain does not mean that they know any methods of reducing the levels of discomfort brought about by vibration. This fact simply shows that the workers have basic information.

Presence of symptoms

Workers who worked more than 8 hours

Percentage of workers who say they work more than 8 hrs

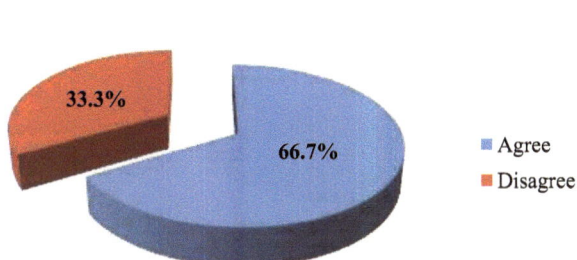

Figure 25: Pie chart showing workers who said they worked more than 8 hours a day.

Although most of the workers agree to the question of working more than 8 hours, it is has to be noted that when questioned about machine operation, the operators and drivers mentioned that they handled the machines for about 4 hours a day. With shifts and job rotations, the sum of all the work done could have gone past 8 hours.

This was not reflected on the day of data collection, as most workers did actually work more or less 4 to 6 hours on the day. What was evident however was that the workers actually worked during weekends.

Percentage of workers who feel pain in lower back after work

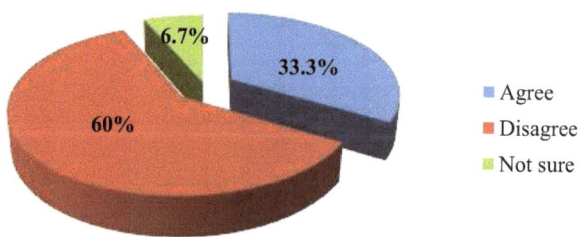

Figure 24. The pie chart shows the percentage of workers who said they felt pain in the lower back after work. Note that 6.7% felt they were not sure

In 1987, Dupuis and Zerlett carried out a study in which 352 earth moving equipment workers with at least 3 years experience were interviewed. 149 workers were asked to rate their discomfort after exposure to 8 hour of vibration. 45% of these workers reported back ache, but this number was increased in the older workers. The authors concluded that long-term exposure to whole-body vibrations causes morphological changes in the lumbar spine (Dupuis and Zerlett, 1987).

Though **33.3%** disagree with the fact that they feel pain in their lower backs after work, it is important to note that only **13%** of the workers that agreed are above the age of 38. This would go in line with Dupuis and Zerlett (1987) study that stated that, the prevalence of back ache increased from **35%** in the younger group, to **67%** in the older group.

Percentage of workers who feel pain in their fingers after work

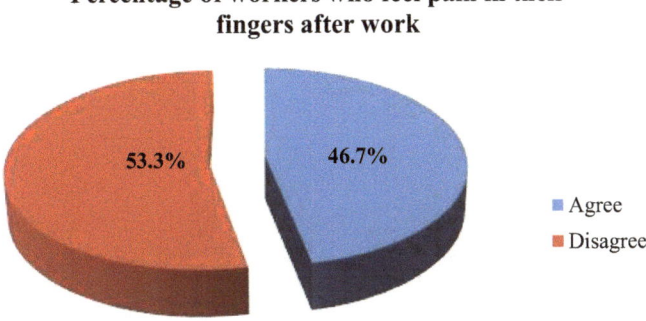

Figure 26: The pie chart shows the percentage of workers who said they felt pain in their fingers after work

It is important to note that the questionnaire was handed to both workers who handle hand help equipment and those that do not with the hope of verifying the presence of a relationship between truck drivers and pain in fingers.

The fact that **53%** of participants disagreed with the fact that they feel pain in fingers after work shows that there is no link between the two. Supporting this is the fact that the **46%** who agree with the question were all hand held tool operators.

The presence of symptoms of vibration white finger could not be verified, as it is beyond the scope of this study.

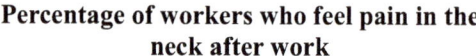

Percentage of workers who feel pain in the neck after work

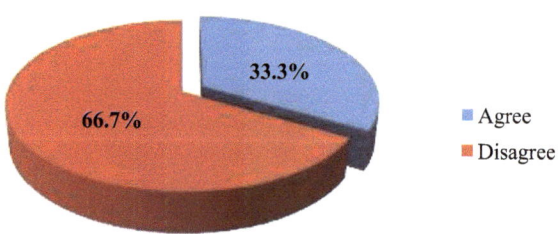

Figure 26: The pie chart shows the percentage of workers that say they felt pain in the neck after work.

Pain in the neck is linked to whole body usually linked with whole body vibration. Zimmerman and his colleagues carried out a study in 1997 in which they investigated work-related musculoskeletal symptoms among 410 operating engineers. About 155 operating engineers responded, and the results showed work related musculoskeletal symptoms in **44%** of the engineers.

The results go against this view, as none of the drivers indicated that they felt any pain in the neck after work. Of the **33%** who agreed, **13%** were compactor operators and **13%** were office workers. This totally goes against Zimmerman and his colleagues, and provides no possible relationship between vibration and pain in the neck.

Workers who complained of discomfort while working

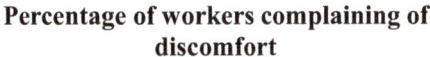

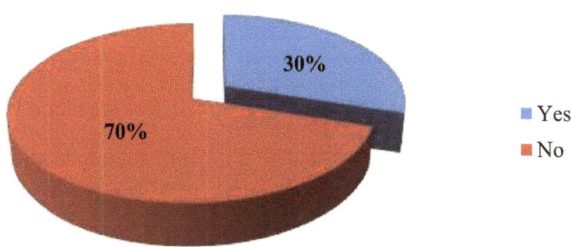

Figure 27: The pie chart shows the percentage of workers who felt discomfort while working

Of the **30%** who said they felt discomfort during work, **13%** were office workers, **and 13%** were heavy duty compactor operators and 1 **(6%)** was a small power tool operator.

This did showed no relationship between discomfort and type of work. Discomfort is a general term that can be caused by a variety of factors. There were probably other reasons for the workers to have felt that they were uncomfortable while working.

6.1.2 Hand transmitted vibration

The daily average vibration values for the screwdriver, the electric drill and the second heavy duty compactor were at **0.0004 m/s²**, while he Light duty compactors (1, 2 and 3) and the first heavy duty compactor had daily average vibration values of **0.001 m/s²**.

These values, when compared to the daily exposure limit value of 4m/s² are very low, which therefore means that the level of vibration transmitted from these tools to the operator through the hand and fingers was will not cause any adverse health effects. There are however several other factors that affect the level of hand transmitted vibration, some of these include:

➢ The magnitude and sustained forces applied through the hands to the tool or the workpiece (e.g. gripping force, axial thrust force, rotational movements)

➢ The orientation and posture of the hands, arms, and body during work (specifically, the angles of the wrists, elbows, and shoulder joints)

➢ The types and sizes of the surfaces in contact with the hands

➢ The total number of years the worker has used vibrating tools on any job

➢ Climatic conditions such as the ambient temperature and humidity and the temperatures of hand-help surfaces of the tool or workpiece.

With this in mind, there may be another factor that may contribute to the development of Hand arm vibration syndrome, such as the total number of years the worker has used vibrating tools on his job.

6.2.2 Whole body vibration

The average daily exposure value for the office worker 2, who was sitting on the standard office chair, was the lowest at **0.049m/s²**. The highest average daily exposure was **0.1141 m/s²** and was recorded by the heavy duty truck driver. Of the two tractors, the heavy duty one had the higher average daily exposure value of **0.0148m/s²**.

All these values are under the lowest level at which one can feel comfortable, which is **0.315 m/s²**. This means that all the participants had no risk of developing any symptoms related to lower back and neck strain caused by high level daily average vibration values.

There also seems to be a relationship between the type of equipment and the daily average exposure values, this is shown below.

Average WBV daily exposure (A(8))

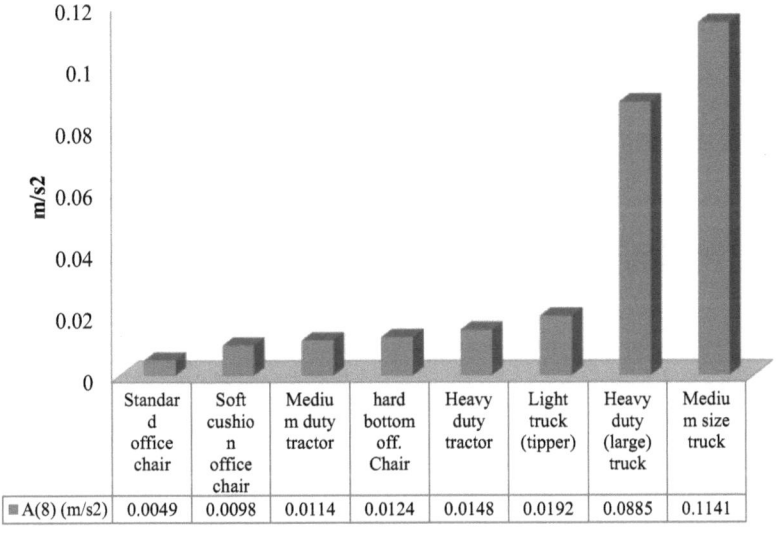

Figure 28: graph showing the comparison of equipment used to average WBV exposure value (A (8))

From the above graph it seems that there seems to be a relationship between the type of chair being used and the value of whole body vibration daily exposure value. There however may be other contributing factors that may induce lower back pain in drivers. Bonvenzi and Betta who investigated the occurrence of low back pain among agricultural tractor drivers (N = 1155) and a control group of office workers in 1994, found that lower back pain was associated with an increase in total tractor driving hours (Bonvenzi and Betta, 1994). Generally, the results seem to agree with Bonvenzi and Betta's study as the office workers' level of vibration was generally lower than those of the truck drivers and tractor operators.

Gustafson-soderman (1987) evaluated the effects of adjustable sitting angle and perceived discomfort in back, neck, and shoulders regions among crane operators. It was found that the highest discomfort values were obtained from operators using ordinary seats. Although standards do not give actual values of vibration magnitude as related to comfort, they do however give some values to which exposed individuals would react to when exposed to whole body vibration.

Table 20: comfort reactions to vibration environments (adapted from ISO 2631/1 – 1997)

Less than 0.315 m/s^2	Not uncomfortable
0.315 m/s^2 to 0.63 m/s^2	A little uncomfortable
0.5 m/s^2 to 1m/s^2	Fairly uncomfortable
0.8 m/s^2 to 1.6 m/s^2	Uncomfortable
1.25 m/s^2 to 2.5 m/s^2	Very uncomfortable
Greater than 2m/s^2	Extremely uncomfortable

The above table confirms that there is a relationship between the level of vibration and the level of comfort, indicating that greater levels of vibration will produce more uncomfortable feeling in individuals. Comparing the results found and the above references, one can say that the level of vibration increases with the lesser quality of the chair. Though this may be acceptable, it is noticed that the medium duty tractor had a lower vibration level than the hard bottom office chair. This may be attributed to the roughness of the road. High levels of whole body vibration are most likely for people who drive vehicles over rough surfaces as part of their job, for example off-road vehicles such as tractors, quad bikes, and dumper trucks (Griffin *et al*, 2006).

7. CONCLUSION

The objectives that were set out at the beginning of the study were achieved. However, the results showed that there was no conclusive association between whole body vibration and lower back pain. Furthermore, the hand arm vibration measurement process was too short; therefore results cannot be confidently used to make any sort of decisive claim.

However, the results suggest that the levels of vibration (both hand arm and whole body) are not high enough to cause any adverse effect to the workers. Furthermore, the daily average values for exposure is lower that the daily exposure limit values, which means that even after daily shifts, there is no adverse health effects from vibration from the machine.

The questionnaire that was distributed assisted greatly in determining the participants' perception of vibration and its health risks, which can be said to be positive, although knowing about vibration does not mean one knows about how to reduce its effects.

8. RECOMMENDATIONS

- ➤ In future, perhaps frequency studies can also be done, as vibration (especially hand transmitted vibration) occurs within a particular frequency range.

- ➤ The study needs a long period of time to be undertaken efficiently, and a large population. These factors could be considered in future vibration studies.

- ➤ More sites could be used, and these could be compared to find out whether vibration levels are consistent. This could be taken into consideration in future.

- ➤ Determining whether the participants are suffering from any symptoms arising from vibration should be considered in future, as it would be an indication that there is a problem, and action needs to be taken immediately.

- ➤ For the above to be carried out, access to medical records would have to be permitted, something that was not allowed during this study.

- ➤ As for the organization, though they have solid administrative engineering controls that insist on job rotation every time one laborer finishes using the vibrating tool, it is also important to educate workers on the importance of personal protective equipment in lowering vibration levels (for hand arm transmitted vibration).

- ➤ Truck and tractor operators also need to be educated in the importance of correct posture and seat adjustment functions in reducing adverse health effects that may arise from whole body vibration.

- ➤ Because of the complaint of laborers, there may need to be a regular internal safety audit that would look into different aspects of safety to ensure that the workers are as comfortable as possible.

9. REFERENCES

1. Bovenzi M., Betta A. 1994. Low-back disorders in agricultural tractor drivers exposed to whole-body vibration and postural stress, Applied ergonomics, Vol. 25, pg. 231 – 241.

2. Bovenzi M., Rui F., Negro C., D'agostin F., Angotzi G., Bianchi S., Bramanti L., Festa G., Gatti S., Pinto I., Rondina L., Stacchini N. 2006. An epidemiological study of low back pain in professional drivers. Journal of Sound and Vibration, 298, pg514-539.

3. Chaffin D., Andersson G., Maratin B. 2006. Occupational Biomechanics, fourth edition. John Wiley and Sons, Inc., Canada.

4. Deboli R., Miccoli G., Rossi G. 1999. Technical Note Human hand-transmitted vibration measurement on pedestrian controlled tractor operators by a laser scanning vibrometer, Ergonomics, Vol. 42:6, pg. 880 – 888.

5. DiNardi S. 1997. The Occupational Environment – Its Evaluation and control. AIHA Press, Fairfax.

6. Dupuis H., Zerlett G. 1987. Whole-body vibration and disorders of the spine. International Archives of Occupational and Environmental Health, Vol. 59, pg. 323 – 336.

7. Eaton S. 2003. Bus Drivers and Human Vibration. Workers' Compensation Board of BC, Engineering Section, Vancouver.

8. Eger T. Whole – body Vibration Measurement. Fact Sheet No. 5 V. 2. Group for Research in Injury Prevention, Laurentian University, Ontario.

9. Frantz R., Holden J., Kielblock A. 1987. Vibration and its effects on the human operator. A literature survey. Chamber of Mines of South Africa Research Organization.

10. Fukanoshi M., Taoda K., Tsujimura H., Nishiyama K. 2004. Measurement of Whole-body Vibration in Taxi Drivers, Journal of Occupational Health, 46, pg119-124.

11. Futatsuka M., Shono M., Sakakibara H., Quan P. 2005. Hand Arm Vibration Syndrome among Quarry Workers in Vietnam, Journal of Occupational Health, 46 pg. 165-170.

12. Gardiner K., Harrington J. 2005. Occupational Hygiene, Third Edition. Blackwell Publushing, Massachusetts.

13. Gracey and associates, 2010. Noise and vibration glossary. [Online: http://www.gracey.com/glossary/glossary-gv.htm#vibration] accessed on the 8th May 2010.

14. Griffin M. 1997. Measurement, evaluation, and assessment of occupational exposures to hand-transmitted vibration, Occupational and Environmental Medecine, 54, pg 73-89.

15. Griffin M., Pitts P., Fischer S., Kaulbars U., Donati P., Bereton P. 2006. Guide to good practice on Hand-Arm vibration, Advisory Committee on Safety and Health at work.

16. Griffin M., Pitts P., Fischer S., Kaulbars U., Donati P., Bereton P. 2006. Guide to good practice on Whole-Body vibration, Advisory Committee on Safety and Health at work.

17. Gustafson-Soderman U. 1987. The effect of an adjustable sitting angle on the perceived discomfort from the back and neck-shoulder regions in building and crane operators, Applied Ergonomics, Vol. 18, Pg. 297 – 304.

18. Harrington J., Gill F., Aw T., Gardiner K. 1998. Occupational Health Fourth Edition, Blackwell Publishing, Paris.

19. HSE, 2005. Control back-pain risks from whole body vibration. Advice for employees on the control of vibration at work regulations 2005. Health and Safety Executive.

20. ISO, 1985. Evaluation of human exposure to whole body vibration, International Organization for Standardization. Ref. No. ISO 2631/1-1985.

21. ISO, 1997. Mechanical Vibration and Shock-valuation of Human Exposure to Whole-Body Vibration. Part 1: General requirements, International Standardization Organization. Ref. No. ISO 2631/1 – 1997.

22. Johanning E., Landsbergis P., Fischer S., Christ E., Gores B., Lurhman R. 2006. Whole-body vibration and ergonomic study of US railroad locomotives. Journal of Sound and Vibration, 298, pg494-600.

23. Kakosky T., Nemeth L. 2003. Musculoskeletal disorders caused by hand-arm vibration, The Global Occupational Health Network, Issue No. 4, pg 3-5.

24. Khorshid E., Alkalby F., Kamal H. 2007. Measurement of whole-body vibration exposure from speed control humps. Journal of Sound and Vibration, 304, pg 640-659.

25. Nyantumbu B., Phillips J., Dias B., Kgalamono S., Curran A., Barber C., Fishwick D., Allan L. 2002. The Occurrence of hand arm vibration syndrome in South African gold mines and the identification of the potential effects of whole body vibration. Safety in Mines Research Advisory Committee (SIMRAC) Report. Health 703.

26. Rahmatalla S., Xia T., Contratto M., Kopp G., Wilder D., Law L., Ankrum J. 2007. Three-dimensional motion capture protocol for seated operator in whole body vibration. International Journal of Industrial Ergonomics, 38, pg425-433.

27. Salmoni A., Cann A., Gillin E., Eger T. 2007. Case studies in whole-body vibration assessment in the transportation industry-Challenges in the field, International Journal of Industrial Ergonomics, pg 783-791.

28. Sampson E., Tonder J. 2006. Development and testing of a screening tool for mine workers with possible hand arm vibration syndrome. Ergonomics South Africa Journal, 1, pg 2.

29. Scarlett A. 2007. Whole-Body Vibration on self-propelled forage harvesters. Evaluation of emission and estimated daily exposure daily exposure levels. Health and Safety Executive.

30. Schust M., Bluthner R., Seidel H. 2006. Examination of perceptions (intensity, seat comfort, effort) and reaction times (brake and accelerator) during low-frequency vibration in x- or y- and biaxial (xy-) vibration of driver seats with activated and deactivated suspension. Journal of Sound and Vibration, 298, pg 606-626.

31. Van Niekerk J., Heyns P., Heyns M., Hassal J. 1999. The measurement of vibration characteristics of mining equipment and impact percussive machines and tools.

32. Vergara M., Sancho J., Rodriguez P., Perez-Gonzalez A. 2007. Hand-transmitted vibration in power tools: Accomplishment of standards and users' perception. International Journal of Industrial Ergonomics 38 (2008) pg. 652-660.

33. www.ccohs.ca/oshanswers/phys_agents/vibration/vibration_measure.html

34. Zimmerman C., Cook T., Rosecrance J. 1997. Operating Engineers: Work-related musculoskeletal disorders and the trade, Applied Occupational and Environmental Hygiene, Vol. 12, pg. 670 – 680.

APPENDIX A: PROBLEM ANALYSIS DIAGRAM (figure is not part of this publication)

1. Consent Form

Title of the study

A study of the daily exposure levels to hand transmitted and whole body vibration of construction workers in a construction site within the University of Botswana

Purpose of the study

To determine the daily exposure levels to vibration of construction workers

- To determine whether the exposure levels to vibration are within acceptable limits
- To evaluate the awareness of workers concerning symptoms related to vibration (lower back pain and hand arm vibration syndrome (HAVS))
- To find out whether the company has any control measures regarding vibration.

Who is taking part in the study

Construction workers and office workers

Risks and/or discomforts

With hand held tools, there may be slight discomfort as the accelerometer will be attached to the index finger, this may cause slight discomfort with long repeated use of the tool.

With whole body vibration, the triaxial accelerometer is placed on the seat. It is designed to make the participant feel as comfortable as possible.

Benefits

The study will determine the levels of vibration on the site, and thus help the company in dealing with any problem related to that.

Voluntary participation

Participation is voluntary and there will be no penalty if the worker refuses to take part

Right to withdraw

The worker has the right to withdraw at any time

New information

Participants will be informed of any new information, so as to allow them to decide whether to continue participation.

2. Questionnaire

Please feel free to answer the following questionnaire, which aims at collecting information on general knowledge of vibration and its health effects. Answers are ranged from a scale of 1 to 5, with 1 being strongly disagree and 5 being strongly agree. Please tick (✔) next to the desired answer.

Part 1:Personal Information

1. Occupation:_____

2. Age range: 18 – 24   _____

                    25 – 31   _____

                    32 – 38   _____

                    39 – 45   _____

                    >45   _____

3. Gender: Male   _____

                Female   _____

Part 2:General Knowledge of Vibration (yes or no questions)

4. Have you ever heard about vibration?   Yes ___   No ___

5. Do you feel comfortable using your tool or while driving? Yes ___   No ___

6. If the answer to No. 5 is no, do you think your tool makes you uncomfortable?

                Yes ___   No ___

7. Do you know the relation between pain in the fingers and vibration?

                Yes ___   No ___

8. Do you know the relation between back pain and vibration?

                Yes ___   No ___

Part 3:Presence of symptoms

1. I work more than 8 hours every day

   1   (Strongly agree)   ___

   2   (agree)   ___

   3   (not sure)   ___

   4   (disagree)   ___

   5   (Strongly disagree)   ___

2. I have pain in my lower back after work

   1 (Strongly agree)   ___

   2 (agree)   ___

   3 (not sure)   ___

   4 (disagree)   ___

   5 (Strongly disagree)   ___

3. I have pain in my fingers after work

   1   (Strongly agree)   ___

   2   (agree)   ___

   3   (not sure)   ___

   4   (disagree)   ___

   5   (Strongly disagree)   ___

4. I feel pain in my neck after working

    1   (Strongly agree)   ___

    2   (agree)   ___

    3   (not sure)   ___

    4   (disagree)   ___

    5   (Strongly disagree)   ___

5. I feel discomfort while I work

    1   (Strongly agree)   ___

    2   (agree)   ___

    3   (not sure)   ___

    4   (disagree)   ___

    5   (Strongly disagree)   ___

FOROMO YA TUMALANO

SETLHOGO SA PATLISISO

Patlisiso ka go amiwa ke dithoromo ga babereki ba kago mo Yunibesithi ya Botswana

[A study of the daily exposure levels to hand transmitted and whole body vibration of construction workers in a construction site within the University of Botswana]

MOSOLA WA PATLISISO

- Go batlisisa kafa babereki ba kago ba amiwang ke dithoromo tsa didirisiwa tse ba di dirisang mo letsatsing.

- Go lebisisa gore a ditoromo tse ke tse di mo selekanyong sese letlelesegang.

- Go lebisisa kafa ba bereki ba lemogang ka teng dikai tse di amanang le thoromo.

- Go batlisisa gore a komponi e na le ka fa e itebagantseng le mathata a thoromo ka teng.

BATSAYA KAROLO

Babereki ba kago le ba diofisi.

BODIPHATSA

Didirisiwa tse di thusang mo dipatlisisong bogolo jang sese tsenngwang mo monwaneng di ka baka gore mmereki a seka a nna sentle.

Sedirisiwa se sengwe sone sese bewang mo setilong, ga se ame ka gope.

BOMOLEMO

Dipatlisiso di tla supa selekanyo sa dithoromo mme se se thuse komponi mo go itebaganyeng le mathata a.

GO TSAYA KAROLO

Go tsaya karolo goa itlhaopelwa, e bile fa mmereki a sa battle go tsaya karolo ga gona ditlamorago dipe.

GO TSWA MO GO THUSENG DIPATLISISO

Mmereki o ka itlhophela go tswa kgotsa go tlogela go ikamanya le dipatlisioso ka nako nngwe le nngwe e a e tlhophang.

DIKITSISO TSE DISHA

Batsaya karolo bat la bolelelwa dikitsiso tse di sha fa dile teng , gore ba tlhophe gore ba tswelela le dipatlisiso kana jang.

SEPHIRI

Maina a batsaya karolo gaana go bolelwa. Melaetsa ee tswang go batsaya karolo e tla nna sephiri sa Yunibesithi ya Botswana le ba Lephata la Botsogo (Ministry of health).

1. POTSOLOTSO

Tswee tswee phuthuloga go araba dipotso tse di latelang, tse maikaelelo a tsone e leng go batlisisa kitso ya gago ka dithoromo (vibrations) le bodiphatsa ja tsone mo botsogong. Dikarabo di rulagantswe from 1 go ya go 5, 1 e leng go sa dumalana tota, 5 e leng go dumalana tota. Tswee tswee tshwaya go bapa le karabo e oe tlhophang.

Karolo ya ntlha: Ka ga wena

1. O bereka o le eng? _____
2. Dingwaga   18 – 24   _____

    25 – 31   _____

    32 – 38   _____

    39 – 45   _____

    >45   _____

3. Bong   Monna   _____

    Mosadi   _____

Karolo ya Bobedi (Kitso ka dithoromo, dipotso tsa ee kana nyaa)

4. A o kile wa utlwa ka dithoromo?

    Ee____   Nyaa___

5. A o ikutlwa o siame fa o dirisa didirisiwa tsa gago kana fa o kgweetsa?

    Ee_____   Nyaa ___

6. Fa o arabile nyaa fa go No.5, a o akanya gore didirisiwa tsa gago di dira gore o seka wa nna sentle?

    Ee_____   Nyaa _____

7. A o itse go amana ga botlhoko mo menwane le dithoromo?

Ee_____   Nyaa_____

8. Ao itse botlhoko jwa mokwatla le dithoromo?

Ee_____   Nyaa_____

Karolo ya Boraro : Boleng teng jwa dikai

1. Ke bereka di oura di feta borobabobedi ka letsatsi

   1. (ke a dumalana tota)   ___

   2. (ke a dumela)   ___

   3. (ga ke tlhomamise)   ___

   4. (ga ke dumalane)   ___

   5. (ga ke dumalane tota)   ___

2. Ke na le ditlhabi mo mokwatleng morago ga tiro ya letsatsi

   1. (ke a dumalana tota)   ___

   2. (ke a dumela)   ___

   3. (ga ke tlhomamise)   ___

   4. (ga ke dumalane)   ___

   5. (ga ke dumalane tota)   ___

3. Ke na le botlhoko kgotsa ditlhabi mo menwaneng morago ga tiro ya letsatsi

   1. (ke a dumalana tota)   ___

   2. (ke a dumela)   ___

   3. (ga ke tlhomamise)   ___

   4. (ga ke dumalane)   ___

5. (ga ke dumalane tota) ___

4. Ke ikutlwa ken a le ditlhabi mo molaleng morago ga tiro ya letsatsi

    1. (ke a dumalana tota) ___

    2. (ke a dumela) ___

    3. (ga ke tlhomamise) ___

    4. (ga ke dumalane) ___

    5. (ga ke dumalane tota) ___

5. Ke ikutlwa ke sa nne kgotsa wela sentle fa ke bereka

    1. (ke a dumalana tota) ___

    2. (ke a dumela) ___

    3. (ga ke tlhomamise) ___

    4. (ga ke dumalane) ___

    5. (ga ke dumalane tota) ___

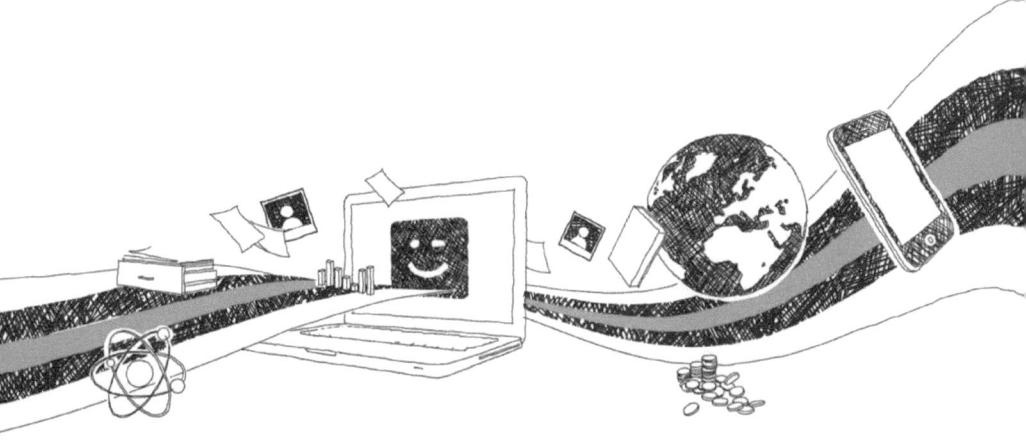
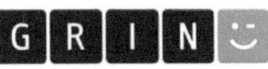